Physician Education Debt and the Cost to Attend Medical School

2020 Update

James "Jay" Youngclaus
Julie A. Fresne

October 2020

Association of American Medical Colleges
Washington, D.C.

This is a publication of the AAMC (Association of American Medical Colleges). The AAMC serves and leads the academic medicine community to improve the health of all. aamc.org

This report was produced by the staff of the Office of Student Financial Services, which helps members of the academic medicine community navigate the complexities of financial aid, student debt, and money management. For more information, contact FIRST@aamc.org or visit aamc.org/first.

Suggested citation: Youngclaus J, Fresne JA. *Physician Education Debt and the Cost to Attend Medical School: 2020 Update*. Washington, DC: AAMC; 2020.

ISBN: 978-1-57754-196-7

AAMC

Contents

AAMC

Acknowledgments

The authors wish to thank the following AAMC staff for their review of and comments on earlier drafts of this report: Cindy Allen, Marie Caufield, Caren Clark, Sarah Conrad, Mary Beth DeVilbiss, Michael Dill, Kristen Earle, Anne Farmakidis, Natalie Felida, Toni Gallo, Julie Gilbert, Doug Grbic, Karen Fisher, Denine Hales, Nicole Knight, David Matthew, Mark Mavilia, Collins Mikesell, Norma Poll, John Prescott, Lindsay Roskovensky, Brett Roude, Matt Shick, Elisa Siegel, Phil Szenas, Lindsay Tiffany, and Geoffrey Young.

Executive Summary

This report summarizes the state of education debt for medical school graduates and the attendance costs of medical schools, with a focus on 2019 data. It updates and complements the AAMC report that focused on 2012 data, *Physician Education Debt and the Cost to Attend Medical School: 2012 Update*. Education debt is the sum of both medical school debt and premedical, including college, debt; they are combined because the sum is the amount a medical school graduate must repay. The report is intended to inform interested readers about recent trends across a range of debt and cost topics and illustrate the capacity of medical school graduates to manage their education debt repayment.

Key findings include:

- The median education debt for indebted medical school graduates in 2019 was $200,000, and 73% of graduates reported having education debt.
- The median education debt of indebted graduates has increased, but at a rate only slightly higher than inflation, and has been stable at $200,000 for the past two years. The percentage of medical school graduates with education debt declined from 86% in 2012 to 73% in 2019.
- Since 2012, many new medical schools have opened, and 16 of them have had a graduating class. Graduates of private medical schools continue to be slightly less likely to have debt but typically have higher levels of debt than public medical school graduates. This difference can be key to understanding apparent debt differences between groups of graduates.
- In recent years, across all medical schools, while cost has been slowly increasing, education debt levels have also been increasing but more slowly than cost.
- Gender differences in education debt amounts and in percentage with debt are negligible and not entirely explained by school type.
- The education debt of graduates varies by family income level, and the largest variations are seen only at the highest income levels.
- Race/ethnicity is associated with variations in education debt, which are heavily influenced both by the mix of private versus public schools attended and by how students expected to fund their medical education when they entered medical school.
- Annual levels of premedical debt — education debt incurred before starting medical school — are remarkably stable, as is the percentage of graduates reporting such debt.
- Noneducation debt is uncommon among graduates overall; however, those who are married, have dependents, or both are more likely to have it compared with graduates who are single with no dependents.
- Graduates with both premedical and noneducation debt have the highest average amount of medical school debt, as one might expect. Premedical and noneducation debt totals are almost always much smaller than medical school debt totals.
- Grants and scholarships rarely cover the entire cost of attending medical school. Private schools typically offer more in grants and scholarships than public schools.

- Specialty content along with a graduate's personality and interests, the influence of role models, and the value of work-life balance all have the highest importance in specialty-choice decisions, according to most graduates. Education debt and potential income do not seem to play determining roles in the specialty choice of most graduates. The influence of debt on specialty choice is weaker than 10 other factors, regardless of debt level or family income level. Interest in primary care is consistent across debt levels.

- The Public Service Loan Forgiveness (PSLF) program has been of interest to a third of all indebted graduates, while more than half of all indebted graduates have reported no interest in any type of loan forgiveness program, whether federal, state, or hospital based. Indebted physicians interested in any of these programs reported having higher levels of education debt.

- Comparing a variety of potential repayment scenarios across various specialties, including primary care, leads to the conclusion that any physician can repay any amount borrowed regardless of specialty or where they live, in part due to the flexible nature of federal repayment plans that link payments to income, not to debt levels. The maximum time span for current federal repayment plans is 20 or 25 years, though most repayment scenarios project full repayment in fewer years. The monthly repayment amounts do not preclude investment in other life goals such as home ownership and retirement savings, though each individual's scenario is unique.

This report was prepared mostly before the onset of the COVID-19 pandemic. It is too early to determine the impact of the pandemic on the future education debt of medical school graduates.

As this report was going to publication, data from the 2020 AAMC Medical School Graduation Questionnaire became available, and the median education debt for indebted graduates was again $200,000. As explained in Appendix 1, some numbers in this report might differ slightly from those in other AAMC publications, such as the *Medical School Graduation Questionnaire 2019 All Schools Summary Report.*

Introduction

Each academic year, roughly three of every four medical students take out federal loans to finance their education in that academic year. Each year, those thousands of loans add up to $3 billion. Taking out federal loans is common to many students earning a graduate or professional degree in U.S. higher education, but medical students borrow higher amounts than most.

By graduation, a typical MD with education debt — the sum of premedical and medical school education debt — will have borrowed roughly $200,000 in education loans. On the one hand, that might seem a challenging financial burden at the start of a career. On the other hand, federal education loans for students are unsecured, with no collateral required, no credit checks (except for Direct PLUS loans), and favorable repayment terms, including monthly payments linked to income, not debt levels. Those conditions are far different from the typical home mortgage or car loan.

According to the 2019 AAMC Medical School Graduation Questionnaire (GQ) data, 73% of medical school graduates reported having education debt, a sharp decline since 2012, when 86% reported having education debt.

For most graduates with education debt, the primary source of that debt is medical school debt. The four-year cost to attend medical school for the class of 2020 surpassed $275,000 at over half of all medical schools and exceeded $350,000 at 19 schools. The four-year cost of attendance, which includes tuition, fees, and living expenses for each year of medical school, is the sum of four years of data from an annual survey of each medical school's attendance costs. The cost of medical school can vary by year at the same school. For example, the cost of the third year of medical school is often more than the first and second years due to more months in the academic year, in part because of clinical rotations.[1]

This report summarizes the state of education debt for medical school graduates and the costs of attending medical school, with a focus on 2019 data. It updates and complements an AAMC report focused on 2012 data, *Physician Education Debt and the Cost to Attend Medical School: 2012 Update.*[2] As with the earlier report, this one covers education debt differences by type of school attended, gender, race and ethnicity, premedical and noneducation debt, and grants and scholarships; the role of financial factors in specialty choice; and the economics of repayment given the array of federal repayment plans available.

Both the 2012 version and this one were based primarily on data from two AAMC annual surveys, the GQ and the Tuition and Student Fees Questionnaire (TSF). Education debt data are from the GQ, sent to all graduating medical students, and the cost-of-attendance (COA) data are from the TSF, sent to all medical schools.[3] As explained in Appendix 1, the GQ debt numbers in this report might differ slightly from numbers in other reports using the same data.

This report includes no qualitative data and does not discuss the emotional and psychological impacts of having to repay education debt. For physicians, such impacts are also influenced by the professional requirement, after graduation, of an additional three to seven years of medical training in a residency or fellowship program. During this phase of training, typical stipend amounts are substantially less than what most practicing physicians earn.

The delayed financial gratification facing most indebted physicians is exacerbated by the economics of education debt repayment during residency. During those years, the income-linked monthly loan payments are often lower than the monthly interest that is accruing, a difficult situation called "negative amortization." Fortunately, as shown in Section Seven of this report, compensation after residency is enough for physicians, with rare exceptions, to repay all levels of education debt, regardless of specialty or residency length.

Section One: Type of School and Education Debt

More Medical Schools Since the Previous Report

Medical schools fall into two categories, public and private, based, in part, on whether the school receives funding support from its state government. Since 2012, many new medical schools have opened, and 16 — 10 public and six private — have had a graduating class that completed the GQ (Table 1). As part of the accreditation process, a new medical school will celebrate its first graduating class four years after welcoming its inaugural first-year class.

In general, in any given year, roughly 60% of both the schools and the graduates who respond to the survey are from public medical schools, and roughly 40% are from private schools, with minor variations in some years (Table 1). This roughly 60%/40% public-to-private-school ratio in the GQ data mimics the overall ratio of public to private medical schools and of public to private total medical student enrollment each year.

Table 1. Total, Public, and Private Medical School Counts in the AAMC Medical School Graduation Questionnaire, 2012-2019

Year	Total	Public	Private
2019	142	85	57
2018	141	85	56
2017	140	85	55
2016	136	82	54
2015	134	80	54
2014	131	78	53
2013	130	78	52
2012	126	75	51

Source: AAMC Medical School Graduation Questionnaire (GQ).

School Type Drives Debt Level

Graduates of public and private medical schools have different median debt levels. Private medical school graduates are slightly less likely to have debt, but their debt levels are typically higher than public school graduates' (Table 2). For this reason, this report's comparisons of debt levels across various groups attempt to account for differences in public and private school attendance by group. There are more public medical schools than private ones, and public schools generally enroll more students; since 2016, the overall GQ data have included 61% public graduates and 39% private graduates. Table 2 also shows that from 2009 to 2019, debt has grown at a higher annual rate, on average, at public schools than at private schools.

Table 2. Percentage of Medical School Graduates With Debt and Median Education Debt for All, Public, and Private Medical Schools, 2009-2019

	All			Public		Private	
Year	Public/ Private	Graduates with education debt	Median education debt of indebted graduates	Graduates with education debt	Median education debt of indebted graduates	Graduates with education debt	Median education debt of indebted graduates
2019	61%/39%	73%	$200,000	74%	$200,000	71%	$215,000
2018	61%/39%	75%	$200,000	77%	$190,000	72%	$210,000
2017	61%/39%	75%	$192,000	77%	$180,000	72%	$202,000
2016	61%/39%	76%	$190,000	78%	$180,000	73%	$200,000
2015	60%/40%	81%	$183,000	83%	$180,000	78%	$200,000
2014	60%/40%	84%	$180,000	86%	$170,000	82%	$200,000
2013	60%/40%	86%	$175,000	87%	$168,000	84%	$190,000
2012	60%/40%	86%	$170,000	88%	$160,000	84%	$190,000
2011	59%/41%	86%	$162,000	87%	$155,000	84%	$180,000
2010	59%/41%	86%	$160,000	88%	$150,000	85%	$180,000
2009	61%/39%	87%	$160,000	89%	$150,000	84%	$177,500
Compound annual growth rate of median education debt, 2009-2019			2.30%		2.90%		1.90%

Source: AAMC Medical School Graduation Questionnaire (GQ).

Note: As explained in Appendix 1, some numbers in this table might differ slightly from those in other reports using the same data source.

Section Two: Current Trends in Cost and Debt

Debt Nearly Stable Despite Modest Cost Growth

Debt levels for indebted medical school graduates have been slowly increasing over the past decade, at a rate slightly higher than inflation. On average, the median amount of education debt for graduates with debt has increased 2.3% per year[4] since 2009, compared with 1.7% per year for the Consumer Price Index (CPI), a standard measure of inflation. In inflation-adjusted terms, the median education debt amount declined in four of the years from 2009 to 2019 (Figure 1). Furthermore, after adjusting for inflation, the median education debt level in the past five years — 2015 to 2019 — was around $200,000 each year, plus or minus $3,000.

Over the past decade, the median cost of four years of medical school has grown at a faster rate than median debt levels, increasing at roughly double the rate of inflation, with upticks every year, even among inflation-adjusted values (Figure 1). Cost has grown more quickly at public medical schools than at private ones, as seen in Table 3 and Figure 2, though debt levels remain higher among private school graduates. Figure 2 highlights some key differences between public and private schools in terms of cost and debt. Public schools typically receive state support and cost less than private schools, while private schools typically have greater resources for grants and scholarships, leading to a larger gap between median education debt and cost at private schools.

Across all medical schools, cost has been increasing slowly, and education debt levels have been increasing more slowly than cost.[5]

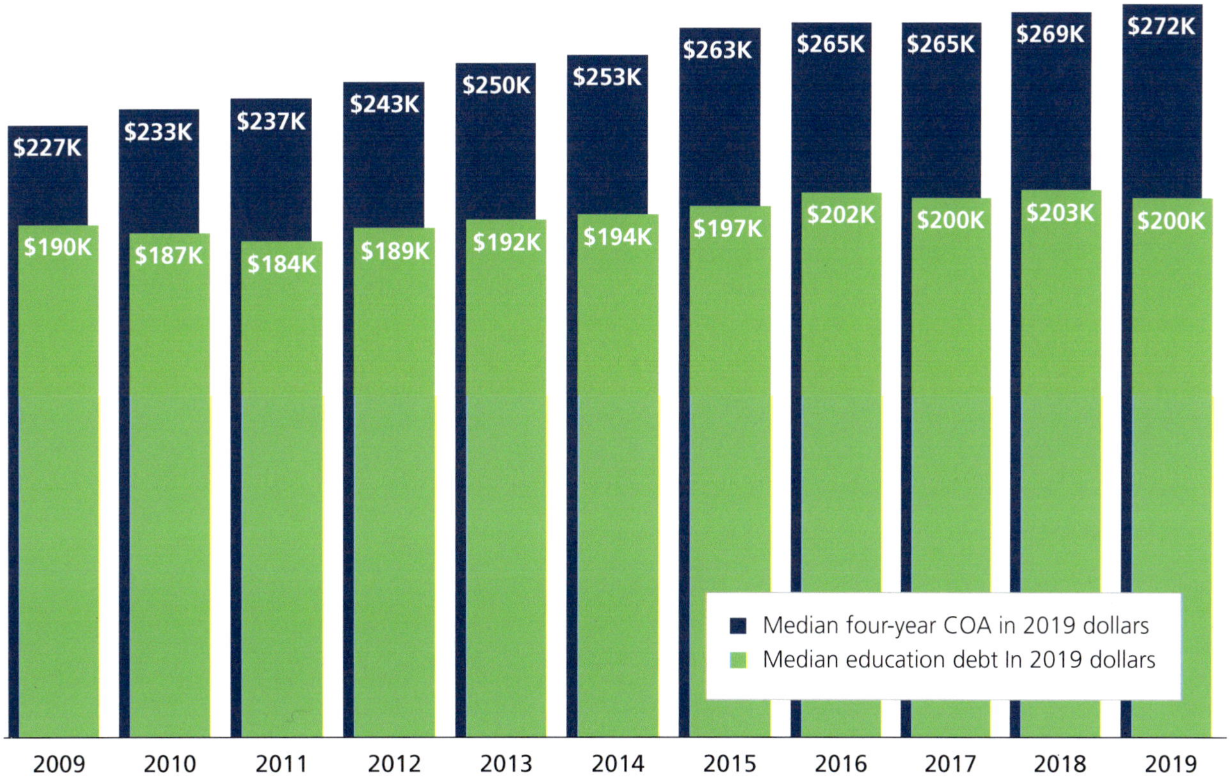

Source: AAMC Medical School Graduation Questionnaire (GQ) and Tuition and Student Fees Questionnaire (TSF).

Figure 1. Inflation-adjusted median education debt levels and four-year cost of attendance (COA), 2009-2019 (in constant 2019 dollars). Education debt = medical school debt + premedical debt. All values are in 2019 dollars using the Consumer Price Index for all Urban Consumers (CPI-U).

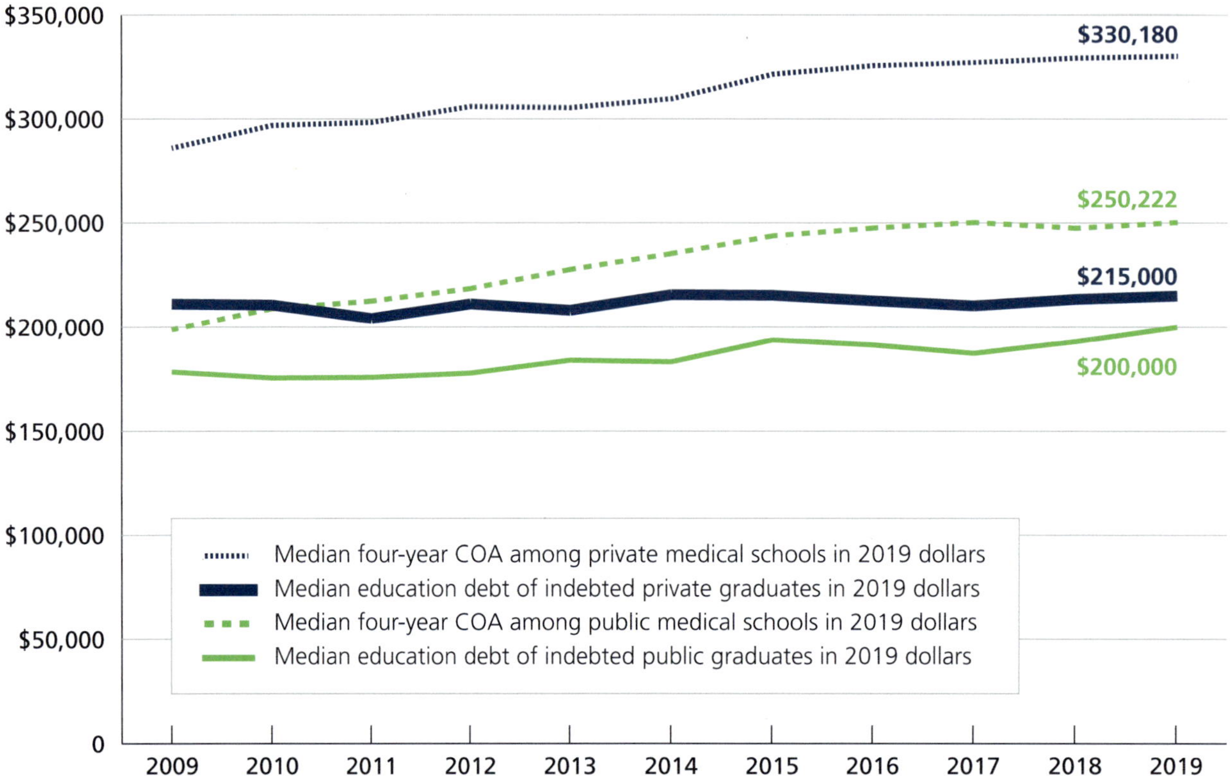

Source: AAMC Medical School Graduation Questionnaire (GQ) and Tuition and Student Fees Questionnaire (TSF).

Figure 2. Median four-year cost of attendance (COA) and education debt of indebted medical school graduates by public or private school, 2009-2019 (in constant 2019 dollars).

Table 3. Median Tuition and Student Fees (TSF), Cost of Attendance (COA), and Four-Year COA for All, Public, and Private Medical Schools for In-State Students, 2009-2019

Year (Public/Private)	Median resident (in-state) four-year COA for graduating class			Median resident (in-state) TSF for first-year class			Median resident (in-state) COA for first-year class		
	All	Public	Private	All	Public	Private	All	Public	Private
2019 (90/60)	$272,429	$250,222	$330,180	$43,151	$38,202	$61,533	$68,924	$62,038	$84,516
2018 (89/57)	$264,825	$243,537	$324,039	$41,400	$36,817	$59,466	$67,195	$60,808	$82,296
2017 (87/57)	$255,141	$240,351	$314,203	$40,654	$36,453	$57,472	$64,622	$59,026	$80,753
2016 (84/57)	$249,368	$232,838	$306,171	$39,716	$35,286	$55,259	$64,023	$57,985	$78,512
2015 (84/56)	$244,801	$226,447	$298,538	$38,939	$34,133	$53,616	$61,866	$56,764	$76,378
2014 (84/55)	$235,120	$218,290	$287,248	$36,604	$33,220	$51,980	$59,750	$55,906	$73,737
2013 (81/54)	$227,988	$207,868	$278,819	$34,966	$32,197	$50,078	$58,556	$53,346	$72,395
2012 (79/54)	$218,510	$196,661	$275,305	$33,736	$30,753	$48,254	$56,565	$51,300	$69,857
2011 (77/53)	$209,468	$187,393	$263,008	$32,176	$28,214	$46,339	$54,587	$49,174	$66,875
2010 (77/52)	$199,474	$178,585	$253,708	$29,962	$26,795	$45,281	$52,056	$48,000	$64,893
2009 (74/51)	$190,721	$167,192	$240,511	$28,253	$24,838	$43,474	$49,807	$44,417	$62,900
Compound annual growth rate, 2009-2019	3.6%	4.1%	3.2%	4.3%	4.4%	3.5%	3.3%	3.4%	3.0%

Source: AAMC Tuition and Student Fees Questionnaire (TSF).

Percentage of Graduates With Debt Declines in Recent Years

Another trend in medical student debt in recent years is the decline in the percentage of graduates with debt (Figure 3). Among 2013 graduates, 86% reported having education debt; six years later, that had dropped to 73%, a sharp decline for a data point that had been stable in the mid-80% range for decades. Flipping the focus of analysis around, the percentage of graduates with no debt nearly doubled, from 14% in 2013 to 27% in 2019, with the largest change in the graduating classes of 2015 and 2016.

While further research is needed to determine the precise cause of the decline in graduates with debt, previous analysis found three factors played a role: the loss of a financially advantageous subsidized federal loan (which had an annual limit of $8,500 for graduate and professional students), a slight increase in the percentage of graduates reporting scholarships, and higher levels of family income (self-reported by medical students as "parental income"). More detail is available in the September 2018 AAMC *Analysis in Brief*, "An Exploration of the Recent Decline in the Percentage of U.S. Medical School Graduates With Education Debt."[6]

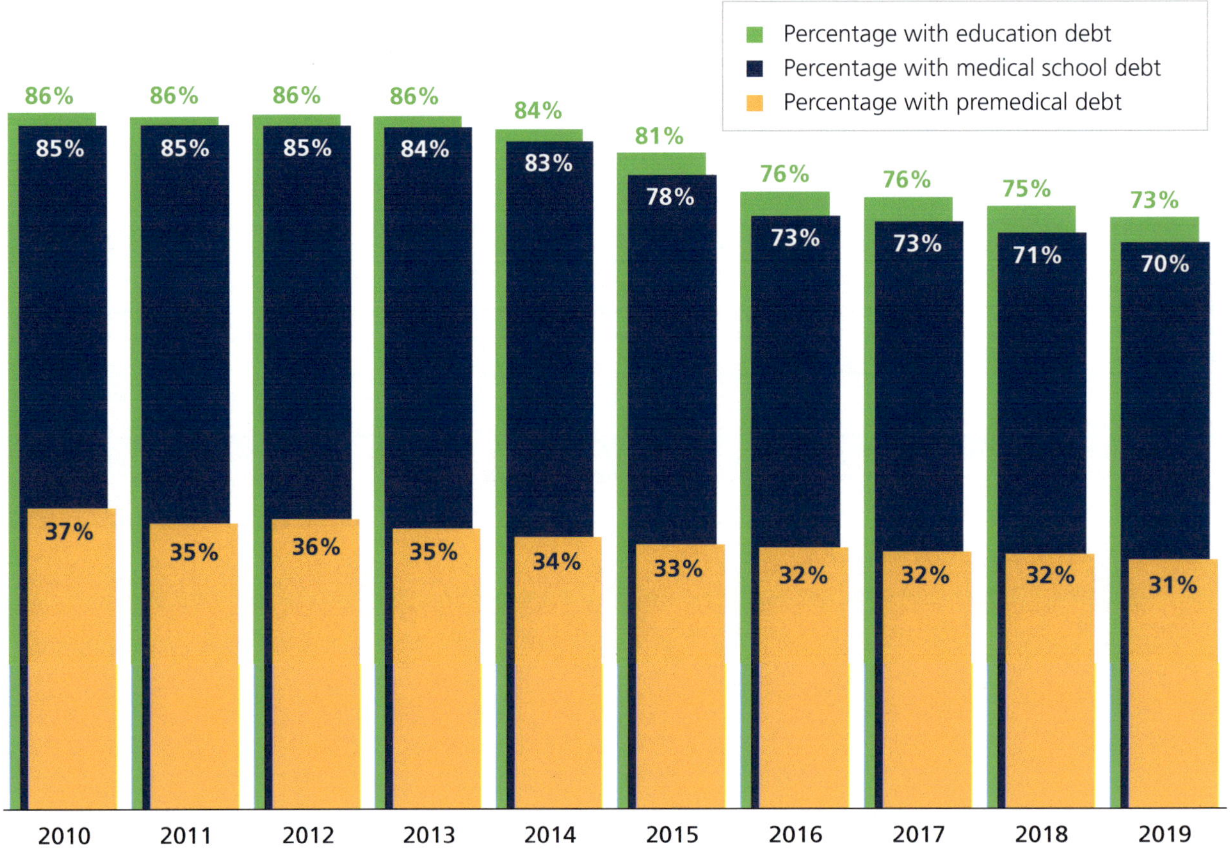

Source: AAMC Medical School Graduation Questionnaire (GQ).

Figure 3. Percentage of U.S. medical school graduates with education, medical school, and premedical debt, 2010-2019. Education debt = medical school debt + premedical debt. Some numbers in this figure might differ slightly from those in other reports using the same data source.

AAMC

Section Three: Education Debt Differences by Demographics

Debt Shows Slight Differences by Gender

In both 2018 and 2019, the median amount of education debt for female and male graduates was the same — $200,000 — and the percentage with debt differed slightly (Table 4). In the years before 2018, female graduates reported slightly lower levels of education debt than males. In each of the four years of GQ data from 2016 to 2019, 39% of all graduates attended private medical schools (Table 2). Over the same four years, 40% or 41% of female graduates attended private schools, while 38% or 39% of male graduates attended private schools (Table 4). Because private medical school graduates are slightly less likely to graduate with education debt but have a slightly higher median education debt level than public medical school graduates, a lower proportion of female graduates with debt might be expected but with a higher median education debt amount than male graduates. However, in 2019, while the proportion of females graduating with debt was lower than for males, as expected, female and male graduates had the same median amount of debt, and in 2018, a slightly higher proportion of females graduated with debt than males — again, with the same median amount. Both 2018 outcomes do not align with expectations based on school type. The reasons for these slight differences between female and male graduates, which are counter to what might be expected based on the proportions of females and males attending public and private medical schools, are not well understood and are worthy of further research.

Table 4. Percentage of Female and Male Graduates With Debt and Their Median Education Debt Levels by Public and Private Medical School, 2015-2019

	All	Female			Male		
Year	Female/ Male	Public/ Private	With education debt	Median education debt of indebted graduates	Public/ Private	With education debt	Median education debt of indebted graduates
2019	49%/51%	60%/40%	72%	$200,000	62%/38%	74%	$200,000
2018	49%/51%	59%/41%	75%	$200,000	62%/38%	74%	$200,000
2017	49%/51%	60%/40%	75%	$190,000	61%/39%	75%	$195,000
2016	48%/52%	60%/40%	76%	$183,000	61%/39%	77%	$192,000
2015	49%/51%	59%/41%	81%	$180,000	61%/39%	81%	$189,000

Source: AAMC Medical School Graduation Questionnaire (GQ).

Debt Stable Across Family Income Levels

The education debt of medical school graduates does vary by family (called "parental" in the AAMC Matriculating Student Questionnaire (MSQ) and "household" in the U.S. Census) income level, but the largest variations are seen only at the highest income levels (Table 5). Other than graduates from families in the top 5% of income nationally, the percentage with education debt varies from 79% to 91% across the remaining groups, and their median education debt amounts are between $200,000 and $212,500. For the 26% of graduates from families in the top 5% of income nationally, more than half — 55% — reported having debt with a median amount of education debt of just over $189,000. The median education debt level for each quintile, regardless of family income level, is comparable to the median for all 2019 indebted graduates of $200,000. Of all the income groupings, the percentage of graduates attending private schools was the highest for graduates with a family income in the top 5% nationally.

Table 5. Education Debt and Other Data by Quintile of Family Income for 2019 Medical Graduates

Variable		Family Income Quintile					
		5th (Highest)		4th	3rd	2nd	1st (Lowest)
		Top 5%: 96%-100%	81%-95%	61%-80%	41%-60%	21%-40%	0%-20%
Family income range		All above $206,001	$112,001-$206,000	$68,001-$112,000	$41,001-$68,000	$21,001-$41,000	$1-$21,000
Percentage of GQ sample		26%	30%	23%	10%	7%	4%
Percentage of quintile with education debt		55%	79%	86%	90%	91%	89%
Percentage of graduates of public or private schools (public/private)		54%/46%	63%/37%	65%/35%	66%/34%	66%/34%	63%/37%
Median education debt of indebted graduates		$189,375	$200,000	$210,000	$210,000	$200,000	$212,500
Percentage reporting medical school scholarship funds		50%	65%	72%	77%	80%	78%
Median self-reported family income		$300,000	$150,000	$90,000	$55,000	$30,000	$15,000
Average for percentage of medical education to be financed with:	"Personal/ parents/ relatives/ spouse/ partner" funds	44%	22%	14%	11%	9%	8%
	"Scholarship with or without a service commitment/ work-study" funds	14%	17%	21%	24%	27%	26%
	Loans	42%	60%	64%	64%	63%	65%

Source: AAMC Medical School Graduation Questionnaire (GQ), 2019, and corresponding Matriculating Student Questionnaire (MSQ). Family income quintiles are based on U.S. Census data.

Table 5 also includes data from the annual MSQ, which has been linked at the respondent level to the GQ data for those who completed both surveys. The MSQ asks students to project how they plan to finance their medical education. They complete the MSQ after receiving detailed financial aid information from their school, so they know both total cost and the levels of institutional and federal financial aid available to them. For this analysis, the MSQ categories have been grouped into three general financial sources: personal/family support, scholarships, and loans. Not surprisingly, as the level of family income increases, the percentage of funds projected to come from personal/family sources rises and the percentage from loans and scholarships declines.

Over half — 56% — of 2019 medical school graduates are from families in the top quintile of U.S. family income, and 79% are from families in the top two quintiles. These results have been similar for more than 30 years. For more information about debt and family income, see the October 2018 AAMC *Analysis in Brief*, "An Updated Look at the Economic Diversity of U.S. Medical Students."[7]

Debt Varies by Race and Ethnicity

Differences among medical school graduates in education debt by race and ethnicity are heavily influenced by whether the graduates attended private or public schools and how students planned to fund their medical education. On the MSQ, medical students project, by percentage, how they will finance medical school. The data on funding sources fall into three general areas: personal/family support, scholarships, and loans. The combination of funding sources and the mix of medical school types attended (public or private) is unique for each racial and ethnic group (Table 6). Key drivers of variations in education debt by race and ethnicity among medical school graduates include school type attended, school location, and funding sources.

Table 6. Education Debt Data for 2019 Medical School Graduates by Race and Ethnicity

						Average for percentage of medical education to be financed with:		
Race or Ethnicity	With education debt	Median education debt of indebted graduates	Public/ Private school	Reported scholarship funds	Median self-reported parental income	"Personal/ parents/ relatives/ spouse/ partner" funds	"Scholarship with or without a service commitment/ work-study" funds	Loans
All	73%	$200,000	61%/39%	62%	$130,000	24%	19%	56%
American Indian and Alaska Native, alone or in combination	80%	$212,375	71%/29%	84%	$90,000	14%	33%	52%
Asian, not Hispanic	61%	$180,000	56%/44%	56%	$120,000	33%	17%	49%
Black, not Hispanic	91%	$230,000	50%/50%	83%	$80,000	8%	34%	57%
Hispanic	84%	$190,000	57%/43%	65%	$70,000	13%	25%	61%
White, not Hispanic	75%	$200,000	65%/35%	61%	$150,000	24%	17%	58%
All others, mostly those reporting multiple combinations of race and ethnicity or "other"	71%	$200,000	59%/41%	64%	$110,000	24%	23%	53%

Source: AAMC Medical School Graduation Questionnaire (GQ), 2019, and the corresponding Matriculating Student Questionnaire (MSQ).

The AAMC race and ethnicity identity data are derived from self-reported student-level data and may include multiple races and ethnicities for a given student. The Table 6 data are not intended as a comprehensive examination of the interaction between race and ethnicity and medical education debt, an important topic that is beyond the scope of this report. Rather, they are presented as a snapshot of 2019 data to highlight information worthy of more study. Appendix 2 includes a breakdown of racial and ethnic identity groupings.

Compared with all 2019 graduates, the proportion of graduates identifying as American Indian and Alaska Native, either alone or in combination with other races and ethnicities, reporting having education debt was higher, 80%, as was the median education debt amount, $212,375. The proportion of American Indian and Alaska Native graduates who attended public schools was higher than for all graduates, which should be associated with a lower median education debt level. American Indian and Alaska Native graduates reported the third-lowest median family income level ($90,000) compared with all graduates and the second-lowest average of anticipated percentage of medical education to be funded by personal or family sources, 52%. Some results for American Indian and Alaska Native graduates are a bit contradictory and worthy of further research. For example, attending public school is typically associated with lower median education debt levels, and lower levels of parental income are typically associated with higher rates of financing with loans.

Compared with all 2019 graduates, graduates identifying as Asian, not Hispanic, reported both the lowest rate of education debt and the lowest median education debt amount — 61% with debt and a median debt amount of $180,000 — despite attending private schools at a higher rate. This is a paradox because, in aggregate, private school graduates are slightly less likely to have education debt than public school graduates, but those with debt have higher levels of it, in part due to the higher cost of private schools. One possible explanation for this paradox is that compared with all 2019 graduates, Asian graduates reported at matriculation the highest level of anticipated funding from personal/family sources and the lowest level of anticipated funding from loans, although, on average, they anticipated that nearly half the total cost would be covered by loans. Asian graduates also reported the second-highest median family income of the six groups in Table 6. "Asian" is a broad category encompassing a diverse array of identities, broken down in more detail in Appendix 2.

Compared with all 2019 graduates, graduates identifying as Black, not Hispanic, were more likely to report having education debt and reported a higher median education debt amount — 91% with debt and a median debt of $230,000. This result is heavily influenced by a higher percentage of these students attending private medical schools, which typically have higher debt levels than public schools. Relative to most other groups in Table 6, Black graduates reported the second-lowest level of family income and the lowest average for percentage of medical education projected to be financed by personal/family sources. All these results mirror the results found for Black graduates in 2012.

Compared with all 2019 graduates, the proportion of graduates identifying as Hispanic who have education debt is slightly higher — 84% — and the median amount of debt is slightly lower, $190,000. Hispanic graduates reported the lowest median family income ($70,000) and the highest average for anticipated percentage of medical education to be financed with loans, 61%. These somewhat conflicting results, where several factors might suggest a higher level of education debt but the median debt level was below that of all graduates, are explained in part by geography and the public-private mix of schools attended. For example, roughly 30% of all Hispanic graduates identify as Mexican American, and more than half of these Mexican American graduates attend a medical school in one of the four states bordering Mexico (California, Arizona, New Mexico, and Texas). Most of the medical schools in this region are public, and public schools typically cost less than private ones. Texas medical schools have attendance costs ranking near the bottom of all schools. Another 26% of all Hispanic graduates identified as Puerto Rican, and 79% of the Puerto Rican graduates attended one of the four Puerto Rican medical schools, all of which have a four-year COA well below the median. The University of Puerto Rico School of Medicine had the most Puerto Rican graduates — 34% of all Puerto Rican graduates — and the lowest four-year COA of all medical schools for the class of 2019.

Compared with all 2019 graduates, the percentage of graduates identifying as White, not Hispanic, who reported having education debt was slightly higher, 75%, and the median education debt amount was identical, $200,000. The proportion of White graduates attending public medical schools was slightly higher, 65%, compared with all graduates, and White graduates had the highest median parental income, $150,000. The average percentage of medical school funding from personal or family sources was 24% for White graduates, identical to that of all graduates, and from loans, 58%, slightly higher than the average percentage from loans for all graduates, 56%.

Section Four: Premedical and Noneducation Debt

Premedical Debt Stable Annually but Varies by Family Income and by Race and Ethnicity

As was the case in the previous version of this report, premedical debt — education debt incurred before starting medical school — was both stable over time and much lower than medical school debt. In each of the past five years of GQ data, 9% of the total amount of all education debt was premedical debt, and 91% was medical school debt. Roughly one-third of medical school graduates reported having premedical debt, and the median premedical debt amount was exactly $25,000 in each of the past four years. Private medical school graduates are slightly less likely to report having premedical debt than public school graduates, but the median premedical debt for private graduates is equal to or slightly more than that of public graduates (Table 7).

Table 7. Percentage of Medical School Graduates With Premedical Debt and Median Premedical Debt Amount for All, Public, and Private Medical Schools, 2015-2019

	All		Public		Private	
Year	With premedical debt	Indebted graduates' median premedical debt	With premedical debt	Indebted graduates' median premedical debt	With premedical debt	Indebted graduates' median premedical debt
2019	31%	$25,000	31%	$25,000	30%	$27,000
2018	32%	$25,000	32%	$25,000	30%	$25,000
2017	32%	$25,000	33%	$25,000	30%	$25,000
2016	32%	$25,000	34%	$22,000	30%	$25,000
2015	33%	$24,000	33%	$22,000	32%	$25,000

Source: AAMC Medical School Graduation Questionnaire (GQ).

Note: As explained in Appendix 1, some numbers in this table might differ slightly from those in other reports using the same data source.

These data are well aligned with the results from another AAMC annual survey, the Post-MCAT® Questionnaire (PMQ), sent to everyone who takes the Medical College Admission Test® (MCAT®) whether they eventually apply to medical school or not. The PMQ asks how premedical education costs were paid, and the 2019 data showed that 41% of these costs were paid from family or personal sources, nearly 40% from scholarships/work-study, and nearly 18% from loans.[8] In general, most medical school graduates were not heavily reliant on loans to finance their premedical education costs.

Table 8 examines premedical debt by family income level. While the median premedical debt amount is similar for each quintile, the percentage with premedical debt varies considerably, with unsurprising trends: The higher the income level, the less likely graduates are to have premedical debt.

The premedical debt of 2019 medical school graduates also differed by race and ethnicity. Among Asian, not Hispanic, graduates, 21% reported having premedical debt with a median premedical debt amount of $22,500. Among Black, not Hispanic, graduates, 58% reported having premedical debt with a median premedical debt amount of $30,000. Among Hispanic graduates, 38% reported premedical debt with a median premedical debt amount of $22,000. Among American Indian and Alaska Native graduates, either alone or in combination with other races and ethnicities, 40% reported premedical debt with a median premedical debt amount of $35,000. Among White, not Hispanic, graduates, 31% reported premedical debt with a median premedical debt amount of $25,000.

Table 8. Percentage of 2019 Medical School Graduates With Premedical Debt and Median Premedical Debt Amount by Quintile of Family Income

Quintile of U.S. Income	Sample in this family income quintile	With premedical debt	Median premedical debt for those with such debt
1st (Lowest)	4%	51%	$30,000
2nd	7%	49%	$27,000
3rd	10%	51%	$25,000
4th	23%	45%	$25,000
5th, top 81%-95%	30%	30%	$25,000
5th (Highest), top 5%	26%	12%	$27,750
Family income not provided	N/A	28%	$27,000

Source: AAMC Medical School Graduation Questionnaire (GQ), 2019, and corresponding Matriculating Student Questionnaire (MSQ). Family income quintiles are based on U.S. Census data.

Note: In 2019, 42% of GQ respondents either did not complete the MSQ or did not provide family income data.

Noneducation Debt Infrequent and Varies by Marital and Dependents Status

The GQ asks about noneducation debt in five categories: credit card, car, residency relocation loan, "other," and mortgage. As with premedical debt, the data show that having noneducation debt is not common and the median amounts (excluding mortgages) are significantly lower than the median education debt amounts. Table 9 summarizes the noneducation debt for each category of debt and includes the sum of the amounts in the four nonmortgage categories.

In the 2019 GQ data, only 18% of graduates — or one in six — had any of the four nonmortgage types of noneducation debt. Among the four nonmortgage categories, while numerous combinations are possible (Yes or No across four categories), four combinations encompass 87% of everyone in the subset of graduates with noneducation debt: 45% reported having credit card debt only, 18% reported having car debt only, 17% reported having both credit card and car debt, and 7% reported having both credit card and residency relocation debt. All other possible combinations occurred less than 3% of the time. The values for each of those four combinations were almost exactly the same in the 2018 data.

Looking further at the characteristics of people with nonmortgage, noneducation debt, an interesting pattern emerges: This debt is more common among the subset of graduates who are married or have dependents. While the GQ question on marital status includes six options, nearly all respondents answered either single (75%) or married (23%). Table 10 separates all graduates into four groups based on marital status and whether they have dependents and shows that the resulting four groups vary significantly in size, percentage who have noneducation debt, percentage of all nonmortgage, noneducation debt they hold, their levels of education debt, their gender split, and whether they attended public or private school.

Among the respondents who provided the necessary data,[9] the "single, no dependents" group made up 76% of respondents but had 55% of all nonmortgage, noneducation debt; the "single, with dependents" group was just 1% of the sample but had 3% of such debt. The "single, with dependents" group was slightly more male and much more likely to attend a public school and have higher median education debt. The "married, no dependents" group and the "married, with dependents" group each accounted for 21% of all nonmortgage, noneducation debt, even though the "married, no dependents" group was over twice the size of the "married, with dependents" group, 17% versus 7%. The "married, with dependents" group, with a median education debt of $210,000, had the highest percentage of males of all the groups, and people in this group were more likely to have attended a public school and slightly more likely to have education debt.

Table 9. Noneducation Debt Data for Medical School Graduates, 2019

Type of noneducation debt	Percentage with this debt	Median amount for graduates with this debt
Credit card	13%	$5,000
Car loan	7%	$10,000
Residency relocation loan	3%	$10,000
Other debt	1%	$9,000
Sum of all four nonmortgage debt categories	18%	$10,000
Mortgage	4%	$150,000

Source: AAMC Medical School Graduation Questionnaire (GQ), 2019.

Note: The percentage values were rounded off.

Table 10. Percentage of Selected Debt Characteristics of 2019 Graduates by Marital and Dependents Status

	No Dependents (93%)		With Dependents (8%)	
Debt Characteristic	Single (76%)	Married (17%)	Married (7%)	Single (1%)
Percentage of all nonmortgage, noneducation debt held	55%	21%	21%	3%
Percentage with nonmortgage, noneducation debt	15%	21%	37%	43%
Median nonmortgage, noneducation debt	$8,000	$10,000	$15,000	$15,500
Percentage of females/males	52%/48%	49%/51%	31%/69%	44%/56%
Percentage graduating from public/private medical schools	58%/42%	69%/31%	70%/30%	73%/27%
Percentage of group with education debt	72%	75%	77%	91%
Median education debt of indebted graduates	$200,000	$200,000	$210,000	$250,000

Source: AAMC Medical School Graduation Questionnaire (GQ), 2019.

Note: Nonmortgage, noneducation debt = credit card + car + residency relocation + other. Single = single (never legally married) or divorced, widowed, or separated but still legally married. Married = legally married, common law, or civil union.

Medical School Debt Amount Varies by Type of Debt Held

When medical school debt is analyzed by type of debt held, an interesting pattern emerges: The average level of medical school debt per graduate increases as the types of debt held increase (see Figure 4). In the 2019 GQ data, the debt of graduates who had only medical school debt averaged $171,000, whereas the average education debt for graduates with both medical school and premedical debt was $212,000. The highest average medical school debt — $229,000 — was for graduates with all three types of debt: medical school, premedical, and noneducation, nonmortgage debt. Note the wide variation in the size of each group of indebted graduates based on the type of debt held. Graduates with medical school debt only were 36% of all graduates; with medical school and noneducation, nonmortgage debt, 6%; with medical school and premedical debt, 19%; and with all three types, 9%. Not shown in Figure 4 are the 30% of graduates with no medical school debt at all, who presumably funded their medical education with some combination of personal, family, and scholarship funds.

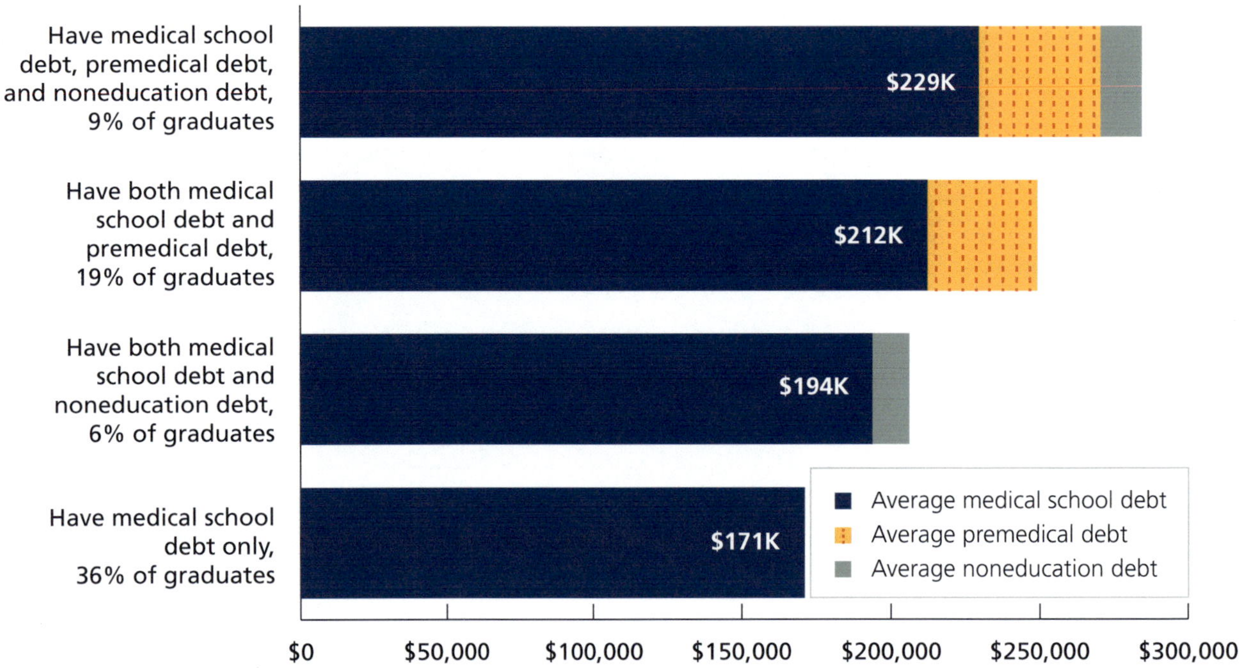

Source: AAMC Medical School Graduation Questionnaire (GQ), 2019.

Figure 4. Average medical school debt by type of debt held, 2019 indebted graduates. Noneducation debt excludes mortgage data and includes credit card, car, residency relocation, and "other" debt. Not shown are the 30% of graduates with no medical school debt.

Section Five: Grants and Scholarships

Grants and Scholarships Are Common but Rarely Cover Entire Cost

Almost two-thirds of medical school graduates in 2019 received grants and scholarships from their institution or from other sources that helped finance their medical education. Few received a "full-ride" scholarship, which covers all costs and allows a student to graduate with no debt.

The analysis in this section, and this section only, includes graduates pursuing an MD degree only; dual-degree graduates are excluded because their scholarship totals can be skewed by the relatively small number of MD-PhD students, who usually receive generous scholarships during their lengthy course of study. For example, in the overall 2019 GQ data, MD-PhD graduates made up just 4% of all scholarship recipients but received 18% of all scholarship dollars. "MD only" graduates made up 90% of recipients, and they received 75% of all scholarship dollars reported by graduates in the survey. The scholarship analysis also excludes graduates of the Uniformed Services University of the Health Sciences F. Edward Hébert School of Medicine, which offers a free medical education in exchange for a postgraduation military service commitment.

The scholarship data in Tables 11 and 12 are remarkably similar to the 2012 data, except the debt amounts in 2019 are larger than they were seven years ago. Graduates of public medical schools in 2019 were still slightly more likely to have received a scholarship than were private school graduates, but their debt amounts were still lower compared with private school graduates. In 2019, private school graduates accounted for 52% of all scholarship dollars but only 37% of scholarship recipients, and public school graduates accounted for 48% of all scholarship dollars but 63% of scholarship recipients. Four-year scholarship totals of at least $100,000 — or $25,000 per year — were uncommon; just 12% of public school graduates and 27% of private school graduates reported receiving such amounts, and even among these recipients, the median education debt amounts were six figures. Recent high-profile announcements about generous scholarship programs at some medical schools might change these numbers in the future.

Table 11. Scholarship Data for 2019 Medical School Graduates Pursuing an MD Degree Only by Type of Medical School Attended

School Type	Graduates reporting scholarship funds	Median four-year scholarship amount among those reporting scholarship funds	Percentage of graduates with total four-year scholarship funds >$100,000	Percentage of graduates reporting scholarship funds who attended this school type	Percentage of all four-year scholarship funds reported by graduates who attended this school type
All	62%	$20,000	18%	100%	100%
Public	63%	$16,000	12%	63%	48%
Private	60%	$40,000	27%	37%	52%

Source: AAMC Medical School Graduation Questionnaire (GQ), 2019.

Table 12. Scholarship Data for 2019 Medical School Graduates Pursuing an MD Degree Only by Type of Medical School Attended and Four-Year Scholarship Amount

School Type	Total four-year scholarship amount reported	Percentage amount reported for those reporting scholarship funds	Median four-year scholarship amount among those reporting scholarship funds	Median education debt for indebted graduates by total four-year scholarship amount reported
Public	None	N/A	N/A	$200,000
	<$100,000	88%	$12,000	$200,000
	≥$100,000	12%	$150,000	$115,000
Private	None	N/A	N/A	$230,000
	<$100,000	73%	$20,000	$248,816
	≥$100,000	27%	$170,000	$130,000

Source: AAMC Medical School Graduation Questionnaire (GQ), 2019.

AAMC

Section Six: Debt and Specialty Choice

Debt Does Not Determine Specialty Choice

Stories in the media about physician specialty choice often speculate that the decision to practice primary care (or not) is governed by some mix of financial motivations that includes education debt amounts, beliefs about future income, and loan repayment concerns. This powerful but unfounded claim persists in academic medicine circles. Surprisingly little evidence supports this assertion, and a comprehensive review of the academic literature yielded numerous research reports indicating little to no connection between specialty choice and economic factors such as debt and income potential.[10]

The GQ data show that physician specialty choice is a complex and personal decision involving numerous factors. Education debt or potential income may play a role when some choose their specialty, but these economic factors do not appear to play a determining role for most graduates. Rather, a specialty's content and its fit with the student's personality and interests, the influence of role models, and the value of work-life balance are the most important factors in specialty-choice decisions, according to most graduates.

Figure 5 shows the influence of various factors on the specialty choice of 2019 graduating medical students. The relative importance of economic factors is clear: Students consistently ranked them toward the bottom of the list, as they have every year for more than a decade. The ranking of the factors, from highest to lowest influence, by 121,000 respondents since at least 2009 has been nearly identical from year to year. Debt and future income do not exert as much influence on specialty choice for most medical graduates as many people think.

What about those with the highest levels of debt? Are financial factors more important in their specialty choice? Figure 6 breaks down the aggregated Figure 5 data into four groups of respondents: those with no education debt and those with their education debt amounts separated into thirds (low, middle, and high). This stratification creates groups similar in size, so each bar represents roughly a quarter of respondents. The two key takeaways from Figure 6 are 1) the ranking of factors was nearly identical for all groups and 2) while those with higher debt amounts were more likely to say education debt had a moderate or strong influence on their specialty choice, it still ranked last for all groups except for those with the highest third of debt, when it rose to next-to-last.

What about those from lower levels of family income? Surely financial factors might be more important in their specialty choice? Figure 7 breaks down the aggregated Figure 5 data into six groups of respondents by family income levels based on U.S. national quintiles of family income; the top quintile is divided into two groups, those from the top 5% of U.S. family income and the rest. The two key takeaways from Figure 7 are 1) the order of factors is nearly identical for all groups and 2) while those with lower family income quintiles were more likely to say education debt had a moderate or strong influence on their specialty choice, it still ranks last for all groups.

What about their actual specialty choices? The GQ asks a two-part question about graduates' "intended area of practice" and specific "subspecialty," if applicable. These data can be compared across debt levels to see how debt levels and specialty choice interact. Table 13 displays the results of a cross tabulation of intended specialties by debt levels, where those with debt are grouped by thirds. Each row shows the percentage and the median debt level for respondents in each cross-section. Data for graduates with no debt and for all respondents are also included.

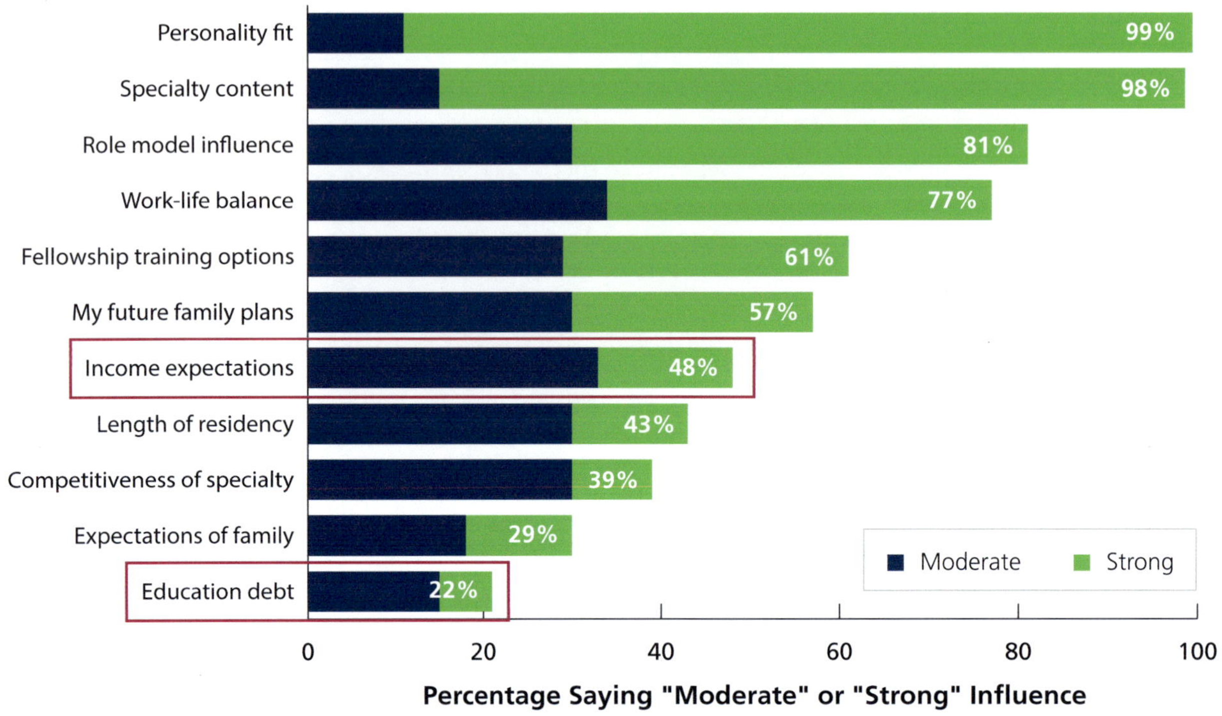

Source: AAMC Medical School Graduation Questionnaire (GQ), 2019, Q32.

Figure 5. Influence of various factors on the specialty choice of 2019 graduating medical students. Boxes surround the two financial factors.

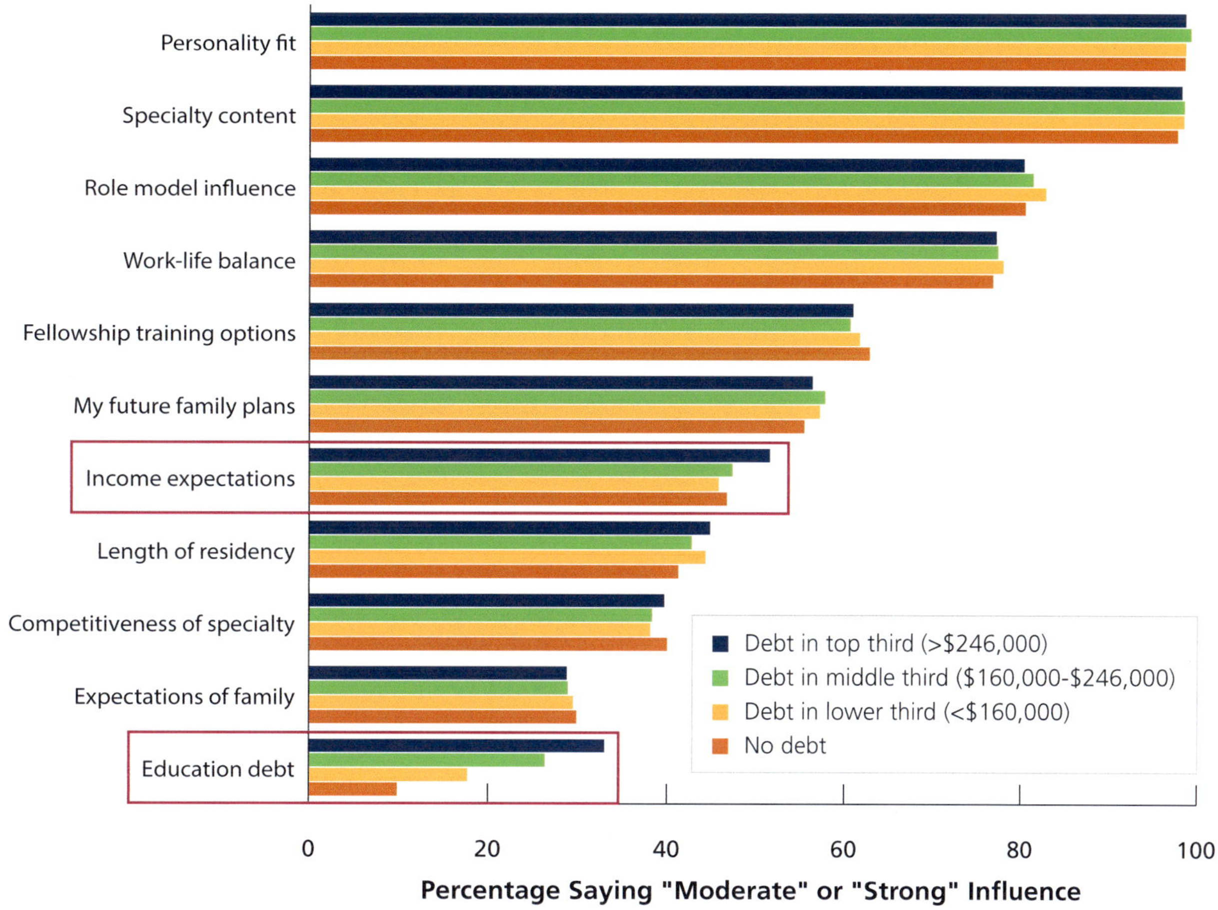

Source: AAMC Medical School Graduation Questionnaire (GQ), 2019, Q32.

Figure 6. Influence of various factors on the specialty choice of 2019 graduating medical students by education debt level. Each debt group is roughly 25% of all respondents. Boxes surround the two financial factors.

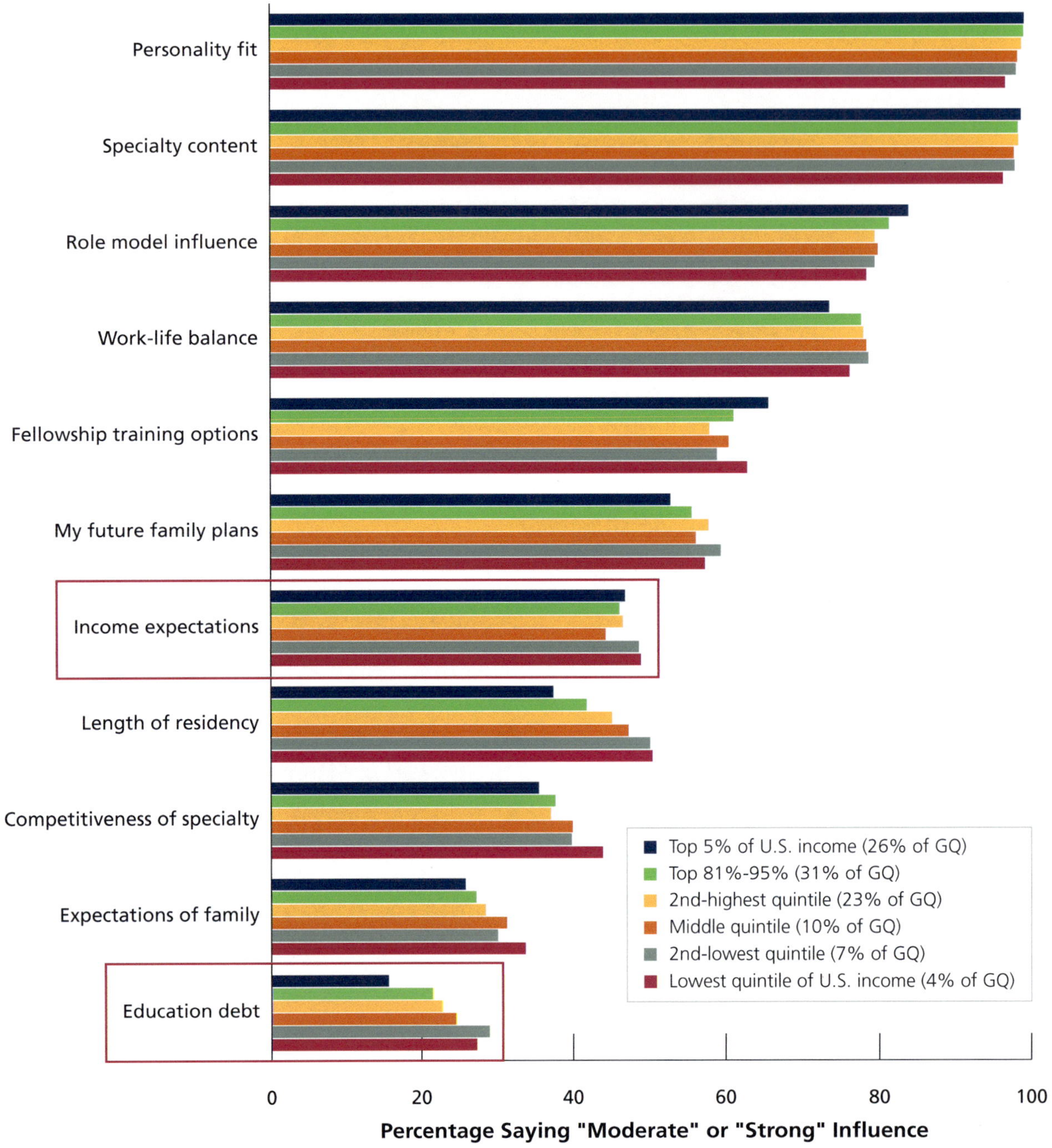

Source: AAMC Medical School Graduation Questionnaire (GQ), 2019, Q32, and Matriculating Student Questionnaire (MSQ).

Figure 7. Influence of various factors on the specialty choice of 2019 graduating medical students by family income level. Boxes surround the two financial factors.

Table 13. Specialty Choices by Debt Level for 2019 Graduates

Specialty Grouping	With Education Debt						Without Education Debt	All Respondents
	<$160,000 (lower third)		$160,000-$246,000 (middle third)		>$246,000 (top third)			
	Percentage of this debt category	Median education debt	Percentage of this debt category	Median education debt	Percentage of this debt category	Median education debt	Percentage of this debt category	Percentage of all respondents
Surgical specialties	16%	$100,000	17%	$200,000	18%	$300,000	17%	17%
Nonsurgical specialties	43%	$97,750	41%	$200,000	44%	$300,000	44%	43%
Subspecialty of internal medicine (IM)	15%	$100,000	15%	$200,000	13%	$300,000	19%	16%
Subspecialty of pediatrics	7%	$96,000	8%	$200,000	7%	$300,000	7%	7%
Primary care: all family medicine, IM and pediatrics, and IM or pediatrics with no subspecialty	18%	$100,000	19%	$200,000	17%	$295,000	13%	17%
Total percentage and median debt	100%	$100,000	100%	$200,000	100%	$300,000	100%	100%

Source: AAMC Medical School Graduation Questionnaire (GQ).

Note: Total percentages might not equal 100% due to rounding. Specialty choice is asked in two parts, first about "intended area of practice" and then about "a specific subspecialty, if applicable." Those selecting internal medicine or pediatrics, "undecided," or no answer for subspecialty were grouped with the respective "subspecialty of" category (i.e., not included with primary care).

Table 13 does not show a bias away from choosing a primary care area of practice for graduates with the highest levels of education debt. Rather, the table reveals quite stable specialty choices within several broad specialty groupings. Graduates appear to have very similar interest in the general specialty groupings regardless of debt level, and the median education debt amount for each grouping within the debt levels by thirds is remarkably similar. Graduates with no education debt show similar levels of interest in each broad specialty group, despite their slightly lower interest in general primary care.

Section Seven: Loan Forgiveness and Repayment Scenarios

Less Than Half of All Indebted Graduates Plan to Enter Any Loan Forgiveness Program

Numerous loan forgiveness programs with a variety of eligibility criteria exist at all levels — federal, state, and local. Since 2010, the GQ has tracked interest in such programs. In each of the four years from 2016 through 2019, while more than half of all indebted graduates reported no plans to enter such a program, a third of all indebted graduates were interested in one program, Public Service Loan Forgiveness (PSLF). Among 2019 graduates, 56% reported no plans to enter a loan forgiveness program and 34% reported planning to pursue PSLF.

The intention of PSLF, introduced in 2008, is to help nonprofits and government agencies recruit employees by promising forgiveness, or cancellation, of all remaining federal student loan balances after 10 years' worth of payments made while employed by such entities, regardless of the employee's profession. Of particular appeal to physicians with debt is that 1) their time in residency or fellowship counts as part of the 10 years if they made regular monthly payments during those years and their employer was a nonprofit, which most teaching hospitals are, and 2) postresidency, they could continue in a nonprofit for the remaining payment years, perhaps by working in academic medicine. The details and regulations about PSLF and how it might apply to physicians are beyond the scope of this report.[11] This brief description merely outlines why many indebted physicians would be interested in this program, which all federal education loan borrowers are eligible to apply for, not only physicians.

As Figure 8 shows, since 2010, indebted graduating physicians have shown rapid, increasing interest in PSLF that has leveled off at a third of them in recent years. The two other forgiveness programs with a notable level of interest, a combined 8% in 2019, include hospital programs with a signing bonus and state-level programs that typically offer some forgiveness in return — for example, for practicing in a rural or medically underserved area of the state. The federal National Health Service Corps (NHSC) appeals to a small but consistent number of indebted physicians who support the program's mission of bringing primary care and other health services to health professional shortage areas. Other federal loan repayment and forgiveness programs include those in the Indian Health Service, the National Institutes of Health, branches of the armed services, and the Department of Veterans Affairs (VA).

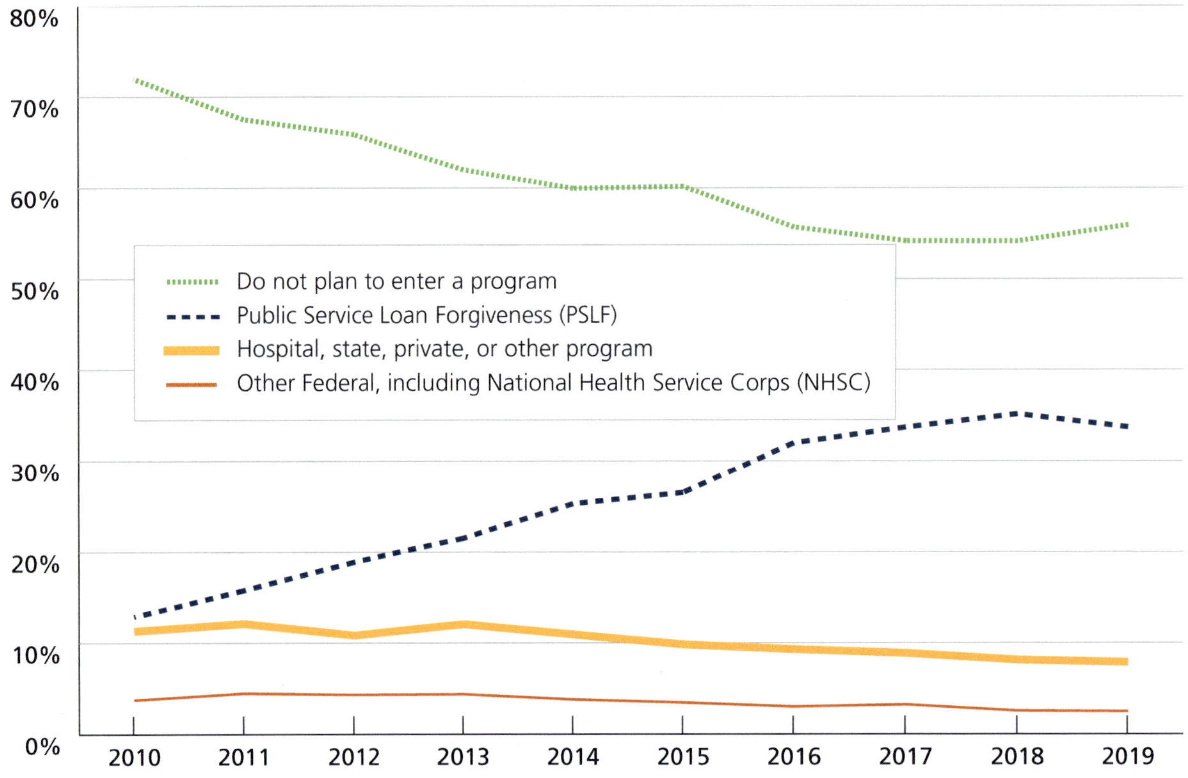

Source: AAMC Medical School Graduation Questionnaire (GQ).

Figure 8. Percentage of indebted graduates interested in a loan forgiveness program, 2010-2019. The "Other Federal" category includes the National Health Service Corps (NHSC), the Indian Health Service Corps, the armed services (Navy, Army, Air Force), and other uniformed services. Public Service Loan Forgiveness (PSLF) is a federal program of the Department of Education.

As Table 14 shows, in general, indebted physicians interested in any of the loan forgiveness programs have higher levels of debt than indebted physicians who are not interested in them. The median education debt amount for those interested in PSLF has been 15%-20% higher than for all indebted graduates each of the past five years, while the median education debt for those stating no interest in such programs has been 13%-17% lower than for all indebted graduates over the same time. Among the third of 2019 graduates with the highest levels of education debt, nearly half indicated plans to enter PSLF, while among the third with the lowest levels of education debt, three-quarters had no interest in any program. Among indebted 2019 graduates of private schools, 38% planned to enter PSLF, while the comparable number among public school graduates was 31%. Although that difference is confounded by the "chicken-or-egg question" — private school indebted graduates typically have higher levels of education debt due to higher costs — the difference is likely the result of debt levels, not some other difference in school type.

Table 14. Various Details of Indebted Graduates by Plans to Enter a Loan Forgiveness Program, 2019 Only

Plan to Enter	Percentage of sample	Median education debt	Percentage of graduates of public/ private schools	Education debt level		
				Lowest third <$160,000	Middle third $160,000-$246,000	Highest third >$246,000
Public Service Loan Forgiveness (PSLF)	34%	$240,000	57%/43%	16%	36%	48%
Other Federal, including National Health Service Corps (NHSC)	3%	$200,000	66%/34%	3%	2%	3%
Hospital, state, private, or other program	8%	$220,000	70%/30%	6%	8%	9%
No plans to enter a program	56%	$175,000	63%/37%	75%	53%	40%
Total percentage, median education debt, and overall percentage of respondents in public/private schools	100%	$200,000	61%/39%	100%	100%	100%

Source: AAMC Medical School Graduation Questionnaire (GQ), 2019.

Note: Total percentages might not equal 100% due to rounding. As explained in Appendix 1, some numbers in this table might differ slightly from those in other reports using the same data source. The "Other Federal" category is for the National Health Service Corps (NHSC), the Indian Health Service Corps, the armed services (Navy, Army, Air Force), and other uniformed services. Public Service Loan Forgiveness (PSLF) is a Department of Education program.

Loan Repayment Amounts Vary by Repayment Plan, Specialty, and Training Length

The repayment of the median education debt amount — $200,000 — can be carried out in many ways, with the total amounts and years determined by a physician's specialty choice, number of training years, and choice of repayment plans during and after residency.

To give some context to the financial effort needed to repay the various debt amounts, Table 15 outlines six scenarios and provides the key values for each, including the monthly payment amounts, the total repayment, and the interest cost. The four primary care scenarios have the fewest residency years among specialties, and the other two scenarios have the longer residency training periods of non-primary care specialties. All scenarios assume $200,000 was borrowed over four years of medical school in federal Direct Loans from the Department of Education at the applicable annual interest rates, roughly 6%. For a 2020 medical school graduate, this borrowing would result in more than $231,000 to repay when they enter repayment, due to capitalization of accumulated interest.

Several scenarios include the most common "income-driven" federal repayment plans. These plans, including Pay As You Earn (PAYE) and Revised Pay As You Earn (REPAYE), link the monthly payment to the borrower's income, not debt level, via a formula based on federal poverty guidelines for household size. Unlike a traditional 30-year fixed-rate mortgage, in which the borrower repays the entire amount through identical monthly payments for 30 years, these plans adjust the monthly payment, up or down, annually, based on a borrower's income and end after 20 or 25 years, depending on the plan. Any remaining amount owed after the plan's time frame, such as in Scenario 1, is "forgiven" by the federal government, meaning it does not need to be repaid, although the forgiven amount is taxable as income.

The financial flexibility offered by such plans, which were first introduced over a decade ago, means that physicians can repay any amount borrowed, regardless of specialty or where they live. To further emphasize that point, the scenarios below include not just the required monthly loan payments but a conservative estimate of the monthly net income, or take-home pay, available to make those payments during and after residency. These net monthly income estimates were derived using an online paycheck calculator that deducts applicable state, federal, and local taxes, withholdings, Social Security, and Medicare, given details users enter.[12] The net monthly income estimates are based on an average of high-, medium-, and low-tax U.S. locations and were rounded to the nearest $1,000.

Scenario 1: Primary care with PAYE during and after residency

In this scenario, a primary care graduate chooses PAYE during a three-year residency and has a $200,000 starting salary afterward. According to payroll calculations based on the national median of first-year-resident stipends, a recent medical graduate, as a first-year resident, would have a net after-tax monthly income of roughly $3,500, give or take a few hundred dollars, depending on location, family size, allowances, withholding, exemptions, and voluntary deductions. The $320 monthly payment estimated for PAYE would seem manageable in this first year and over the next two years, when the monthly payment would increase roughly $25 annually as the resident's stipend increased. Unfortunately for physicians at this debt level and higher, the negative amortization that occurs each month of residency because the monthly payments are lower than the monthly interest that accrues extends the future total repayment time frame by a few years.

After the three-year residency, with a starting salary in line with national compensation data for primary care physicians, the initial monthly payment would be about $1,600, which also seems manageable with a roughly $10,000 net after-tax monthly income (based on a pretax $200,000 annual income). That monthly payment would increase by roughly $35 annually as the physician's income increases 2% annually until it reaches a cap in the program's final years, a technical detail unique to the PAYE plan. After 20 years of payments, this primary care borrower would repay the entire $200,000 borrowed, with a total repayment of $416,000 and a remaining balance of about $38,000, which would be forgiven. Since the $38,000 would be taxable, the borrower would more likely choose REPAYE (Scenario 2) than PAYE.

Scenario 2: Primary care with REPAYE during and after residency

This scenario is identical to Scenario 1, except the primary care graduate chooses REPAYE during and after residency. The REPAYE plan offers a 50% subsidy on unpaid monthly interest, which the PAYE program does not offer, making REPAYE likely more appealing to residents with longer residencies or higher education debt. Even with this subsidy, negative amortization would occur each month of residency at this debt level.

While REPAYE results in the same monthly payment amounts as PAYE during and immediately after residency, several years after residency, REPAYE results in a higher monthly payment than PAYE because REPAYE does not have PAYE's monthly payment cap. Because the total of unpaid monthly interest during residency is lower and the monthly payment in later years is higher than it is for PAYE, this primary care borrower repays all their education debt, with a total repayment of $421,000, and no forgiveness, after 20 years.

Scenario 3: Nonsurgical specialty with REPAYE during and after residency

In this scenario, a graduate chooses a nonsurgical specialty and the REPAYE payment plan. The residency lasts four years, followed by a $275,000 starting salary. The monthly payments during residency are the same as in Scenarios 1 and 2 for the first three years, about $320; in the fourth year, they would be about $400. After residency, the higher starting salary means a monthly payment starting at roughly $2,400, which seems manageable with roughly $13,000 in net monthly income (based on the $275,000 annual income). Given a modest 2% annual increase in income, the monthly payments would increase by roughly $50 annually after residency. After 15 years of repayment, 11 of them after residency, all education debt would be repaid, with a total repayment of $364,000. That is less than the total for Scenarios 1 and 2 because the higher monthly payments after residency mean it takes fewer years to repay the debt.

Scenario 4: Primary care with forbearance during residency and Standard 10-year repayment after residency

Graduates needing to maximize their monthly income during residency might consider choosing forbearance, which requires no payments, although monthly interest does accumulate with no subsidy. This leads to a larger postresidency balance to repay. With forbearance during a three-year residency followed by the most aggressive repayment option — the Department of Education Standard 10-year plan — the borrower would have fixed monthly payments of roughly $3,000 and roughly $10,000 in net monthly income in the first postresidency year. The estimated total repayment amount of this scenario is $365,000.

Scenario 5: Surgical specialty with forbearance during residency and Standard 10-year repayment after residency

This scenario is the same as Scenario 4 but with the longer residency associated with surgical specialties. With forbearance during the seven-year residency of this scenario, much more interest would accrue during residency, leading to a postresidency monthly payment of roughly $3,700 for the Standard 10-year plan. However, the physician's net monthly income postresidency would be notably higher than Scenario 4's primary care physician; the starting net monthly income for physicians in most surgical specialties is at least $15,000 in the first postresidency year, a sum that could accommodate the Standard monthly payment. The total estimated repayment amount of this scenario is $440,000, which is greater than Scenario 4's due to the three extra years of interest that would accrue during the seven-year residency.

Scenario 6: Primary care with REPAYE during and after residency and PSLF

The final scenario outlines a primary care physician pursuing PSLF, the program with forgiveness of any remaining balance after 10 years' worth of payments, as described at the beginning of this section. The postresidency starting salary in this scenario is $170,000, reflecting the lower salaries associated with the nonprofit career pathway. The monthly payments in REPAYE are comparable to those mentioned in Scenario 2, projected to be around $1,600 in the 10th year. The projected repayment amount would be $135,000, and roughly $221,000 would be forgiven. This PSLF 10-year forgiveness would not be taxed. This scenario highlights how medical school graduates interested in a public service or academic medicine career need not be deterred by financial concerns related to loan repayment. The federal repayment plans allow for manageable monthly payments during and after residency that seem unlikely to severely hamper household finances given the projected net monthly income during and after residency.

Table 15. Various Repayment Scenarios for a 2019 Graduate With $200,000 in Federal Direct Loans

Scenario	Residency		Postresidency		Interest Cost	Total Repayment
	Repayment Years	Monthly Payment	Repayment Years	Monthly Payment		
1: PAYE during residency and after with $200,000 starting salary	3	$320-$370	17	$1,600-$2,400	$254,000	$416,000, then ≈$38,000 forgiven
2: REPAYE during residency and after with $200,000 starting salary	3	$320-$370	17	$1,600-$2,500	$221,000	$421,000
3: REPAYE during residency and after with $275,000 starting salary	4	$320-$400	11	$2,400-$3,000	$164,000	$364,000
4: Primary care, forbearance during residency, then Standard	3	$0	10	$3,000	$165,000	$365,000
5: Surgical specialty, forbearance during residency, then Standard	7	$0	10	$3,700	$240,000	$440,000
6: REPAYE during residency and after with $170,000 starting salary and PSLF	3	$320-$370	7	$1,400-$1,600	$135,000	$135,000, then ≈$221,000 forgiven

Source: Authors' analyses of federal repayment program details as applied to a medical school graduate.

Note: PAYE = Pay As You Earn. REPAYE = Revised Pay As You Earn. PSLF = federal Public Service Loan Forgiveness program. All figures are approximate, rounded off, and estimated for a 2019 graduate. Salaries are in 2018 dollars. Non-PSLF amounts forgiven are taxable. Custom repayment scenarios can be analyzed by physician borrowers using the AAMC MedLoans® Organizer and Calculator available at aamc.org/FIRST.

Final Note

The previous version of this report analyzed the cost and debt data for the medical school class of 2012. In the seven years of data analyzed since that report, several notable trends have emerged, including:

- The percentage of medical school graduates with education debt has declined from 86% in 2012 to 73% in 2019.
- The median education debt of indebted graduates has increased, but at a rate only slightly higher than inflation, and has been stable at $200,000 for the past two years.
- Federal repayment plans have become more favorable with the December 2015 introduction of REPAYE, which provides an interest subsidy beneficial to residents in active repayment and links monthly payments to income, not debt, level.
- Several medical schools have announced high-profile initiatives to provide significant grants and scholarship funds to all their medical students at levels that will significantly reduce students' education debt at graduation.

Although these trends are favorable to medical students generally, the data continue to show that three out of four students graduate from medical school with education debt, most often with six-figure dollar amounts. The economics of loan repayment indicate that indebted physicians in all specialties should be able to repay their student loans comfortably, though that could take 10-20 years or more, depending on their circumstances. Medical education, while expensive, remains a good investment.[13]

"Medical education has become increasingly expensive, and many students will face the challenges of assuming significant debt during their education. Although the prospect of debt at this level is daunting and may deter some students and families from even considering a medical education, the AAMC will continue to work with students to address this concern with clear information and guidance. The data are clear: For most physicians, future earnings will permit repayment and the achievement of personal financial-planning goals. Medical schools should continue to work to limit the debt levels of their students, consonant with prudent management of their institution."

— David J. Skorton, MD, AAMC President and CEO

AAMC

Notes

1. See Appendix 1 for more details about four-year cost-of-attendance data.

2. Youngclaus J, Fresne JA. *Physician Education Debt and the Cost to Attend Medical School: 2012 Update.* Washington, DC: AAMC; 2013. Available at aamc.org/data-reports/students-residents/report/physician-education-debt-and-cost-attend-medical-school.

3. The 2019 GQ had 16,657 respondents representing 83.6% of the 19,933 medical students who graduated from July 1, 2018, through June 30, 2019. The 2019 TSF had a response rate of 100% from the 151 medical schools.

4. As measured by the compound annual growth rate or average annual growth rate over the time frame, calculated as the geometric average of the annual growth rates during the years of analysis.

5. Youngclaus J, Bunton SA, Fresne J. An updated look at attendance cost and medical student debt at U.S. medical schools. *Analysis in Brief.* 2017;17(1):1-3.

6. Youngclaus J. An exploration of the recent decline in the percentage of U.S. medical school graduates with education debt. *Analysis in Brief.* 2018;18(4):1-3. Available at aamc.org/data-reports/analysis-brief/report/exploration-recent-decline-percentage-us-medical-school-graduates-education-debt.

7. Youngclaus J, Roskovensky L. An updated look at the economic diversity of U.S. medical students. *Analysis in Brief.* 2018;18(5):1-3. Available at aamc.org/data-reports/analysis-brief/report/updated-look-economic-diversity-us-medical-students.

8. See Q16 results in the *Post-MCAT Questionnaire, 2019 Report*, available at aamc.org/system/files/2020-02/2019%20PMQ%20Summary%20Report.pdf. Note that similar categories in the Q16 data have been combined for brevity.

9. In the 2019 GQ, 91.2% of all respondents provided data on marital status, number of dependents, and noneducation debt. The survey asks, "How many dependents do you have (not including a spouse/partner)?"; most dependents of medical students are probably children.

10. See Kahn MJ, Markert RJ, Lopez FA, Randall H, Krane NK. Is medical student choice of a primary care residency influenced by debt? *Med Gen Med.* 2006;8(4):18. Available at pubmedcentral.nih.gov/articlerender.fcgi?artid=1868367. Frank E, Feinglass S. Student loan debt does not predict female physicians' choice of primary care specialty. *J Gen Intern Med.* 1999; 4(6):347-350. doi:10.1046/j.1525-1497.1999.00339.x. McDonald FS, West CP, Popkave C, Kolars JC. Educational debt and reported career plans among internal medicine residents. *Ann Intern Med.* 2008;149(6):416-420. doi:10.7326/0003-4819-149-6-200809160-00008. For a different research approach leading to similar conclusions, see Marcu MI, Kellermann AL, Hunter C, Curtis J, Rice C, Wilensky GR. Borrow or serve? An economic analysis of options for financing a medical school education. *Acad Med.* 2017;92:966-975. doi: 10.1097/ACM.0000000000001572.

11. The AAMC provides a comprehensive array of PSLF resources, with details on eligibility for medical students, at students-residents.aamc.org/financial-aid/article/public-service-loan-forgiveness-pslf/.

12. PaycheckCity at paycheckcity.com/.

13. Prescott JE, Fresne JA, Youngclaus JA. The good investment. *Acad Med.* 2017;92(7):912-913. doi:10.1097/ACM.0000000000001573.

Appendix 1. Methodology

Most analyses in this report are based primarily on data from two AAMC annual surveys, the Medical School Graduation Questionnaire (GQ) and the Tuition and Student Fees Questionnaire (TSF). Education debt data are from the GQ, sent to all graduating medical students, and the cost-of-attendance (COA) data are from the TSF, sent to all medical schools. The TSF had a response rate of 100% in 2019, and the data are publicly available (see aamc.org/data-reports/reporting-tools/report/tuition-and-student-fees-reports). According to information about the TSF on the AAMC website, "The tuition, fees, and health insurance costs are the costs published by medical schools. As a result, these costs do reflect discounts resulting from grants, scholarships, or stipends." The TSF collects data on the cost of each year of medical school for every school, including tuition, fees, and living expenses. The four-year COA is the sum of the cost for a single class at a school over four years. For example, the four-year cost at School X for the class of 2019 was the sum of the first-year COA in 2015-2016, plus the second-year COA in 2016-2017, plus the third-year COA in 2017-2018, plus the fourth-year COA in 2018-2019.

The Medical School Graduation Questionnaire: 2019 All Schools Summary Report (available at aamc.org/system/files/2019-08/2019-gq-all-schools-summary-report.pdf) notes the report's data represent "the responses of 16,657 graduates of the 142 U.S. medical schools that graduated students in the 2018-2019 academic year. According to the AAMC Student Records System (SRS) as of July 8, 2019, these 16,657 respondents represent 83.6% of the 19,933 medical students who graduated from July 1, 2018, through June 30, 2019. Survey data for participating individuals may not be comparable to data for nonparticipants." While most graduates answered all the questions, not all did; for example, more than 15,000 graduates answered the questions about premedical and medical debt, and more than 15,700 graduates answered the question about which specialty they intend to practice, but some answered the debt questions and not the specialty-choice question and vice versa. The numbers of respondents to a given question vary and are not included in this report. Sample sizes are available on request.

The 2019 GQ debt data in this report might occasionally differ slightly from debt data in other reports that use GQ data, such as the *Medical School Graduation Questionnaire: 2019 All Schools Summary Report*. This is because the AAMC Office of Student Financial Services staff applies several additional data-processing steps before the data are analyzed, such as not including premedical or medical debt values less than $1,000. The data-processing steps are available on request.

Data from the AAMC Matriculating Student Questionnaire (MSQ) are used in some analyses. The MSQ is sent to all matriculating medical students when they enter medical school; in 2019, the survey response rate slightly exceeded 71% (for details, see aamc.org/system/files/2019-12/2019%20MSQ%20All%20Schools%20Summary%20Report.pdf). If the same medical student completes both surveys, their responses across the years may be linked for research purposes. The following question is on the MSQ: "Regardless of your dependency status, please indicate your parents' combined gross income for last year (a rough estimate is sufficient)." This information can be cross-referenced, by year, with national U.S. Census data on household-income-quintile values to allow the family income analyses found throughout this report. The MSQ also asks students to project how they plan to finance their medical education on a percentage basis across multiple categories. Students complete the MSQ after receiving detailed financial aid information from their school, so they have been well-informed about both total costs and the levels of institutional and federal financial aid available to them.

Appendix 2. More Detail on Education Debt and Race and Ethnicity

This appendix expands Table 6, Education Debt Data for 2019 Medical School Graduates by Race and Ethnicity. It includes a more detailed breakdown for specific self-identified groups, each of which had at least 20 graduates included in the 2019 GQ data, or roughly 0.10% of the sample.

Table A.1. Education Debt Data for 2019 Medical School Graduates by Race and Ethnicity, Expanded

Race or Ethnicity	Percentage of sample	Percentage with education debt	Percentage from public/ private schools	Median education de of indebted graduate
American Indian and Alaska Native: In Combination	0.70%	83%	65%/35%	$218,000
American Indian and Alaska Native	0.20%	65%	97%/3%	$200,000
Asian	2%	63%	55%/45%	$184,222
East Asian: Chinese	5%	56%	49%/51%	$158,500
East Asian: Korean	2%	77%	48%/52%	$215,000
East Asian: Taiwanese	1.10%	51%	53%/47%	$147,500
East Asian: Japanese	0.30%	52%	57%/43%	$180,000
East Asian	0.60%	55%	55%/45%	$169,809
South Asian: Indian	7%	55%	59%/41%	$172,501
South Asian: Pakistani	0.90%	79%	66%/34%	$199,000
South Asian: Bangladeshi	0.30%	75%	59%/41%	$192,500
Southeast Asian: Vietnamese	1.40%	75%	68%/32%	$186,000
Southeast Asian: Filipino	0.60%	80%	62%/38%	$242,500
Southeast Asian	0.10%	61%	62%/38%	$200,000
Black: African-American	3%	91%	55%/45%	$225,000
Black: African	0.90%	86%	50%/50%	$210,000
Black: Caribbean	0.70%	95%	39%/61%	$255,500
Black	2%	92%	43%/57%	$240,000
Hispanic: Mexican	2%	89%	71%/29%	$192,000
Hispanic: Puerto Rican	1.30%	80%	43%/57%	$175,000
Hispanic: Cuban	0.40%	78%	66%/34%	$203,500
Hispanic: Colombian	0.30%	74%	53%/47%	$180,000
Hispanic: Peruvian	0.20%	93%	60%/40%	$195,250
Hispanic: Dominican	0.10%	89%	52%/48%	$170,575
Hispanic	1.30%	83%	54%/46%	$200,000
Other	2%	69%	59%/41%	$220,000
Multiple races and ethnicities selected	7%	72%	59%/41%	$200,000
White, not Hispanic	57%	75%	65%/35%	$200,000

Source: AAMC Medical School Graduation Questionnaire (GQ), 2019, and the corresponding Matriculating Student Questionnaire (MSQ).

Note: Each group in this table is separate from all other groups in the table, including the more general identity groups such as Southeast Asian, Black, and Hispanic; there is no overlap. For example, the identity grouping "East Asian" includes respondents who identified as East Asian or as multiple East Asian identities, such as both Korean and Japanese. The "Asian" grouping includes respondents who identified as Asian or as multiple Asian identities, such as both Chinese and Vietnamese. The "Southeast Asian" grouping includes respondents who identified as Indonesian only (n = 10), as Cambodian only (n = 9), or as Laotian only (n = 1). The "Hispanic" grouping includes respondents who identified as Argentinian only (n = 8). The "Other" grouping includes respondents who identified as Native Hawaiian only (n = 5) and as Guamanian only (n = 3). The "American Indian and Alaska Native: In Combination" grouping includes respondents who identified as both "American Indian and Alaska Native" and any other grouping; the "American Indian and Alaska Native" grouping includes respondents who identified as "American Indian and Alaska Native" only.

AAMC

Percentage of group reporting scholarship funds	Median self-reported parental income for all in the group	Average for percentage of medical education to be financed with:		
		"Personal/parents/relatives/spouse/partner" funds	"Scholarship with or without a service commitment/work-study" funds	Loans
83%	$85,000	13%	34%	52%
87%	$90,000	15%	27%	58%
62%	$100,000	30%	24%	36%
57%	$140,000	36%	21%	43%
62%	$80,000	19%	18%	62%
55%	$110,000	40%	16%	43%
62%	$190,000	35%	20%	42%
64%	$150,000	33%	19%	44%
48%	$160,000	38%	13%	49%
65%	$100,000	22%	20%	58%
60%	$105,000	28%	21%	52%
66%	$65,000	24%	16%	60%
61%	$100,000	15%	16%	69%
67%	$70,000	14%	16%	71%
87%	$90,000	7%	36%	56%
83%	$60,000	11%	33%	55%
84%	$60,000	4%	34%	62%
78%	$80,500	8%	33%	58%
78%	$65,500	7%	30%	63%
35%	$75,000	18%	14%	67%
70%	$100,000	21%	23%	56%
87%	$72,500	15%	31%	51%
81%	$51,500	6%	33%	61%
70%	$36,000	19%	42%	39%
73%	$70,000	12%	28%	59%
57%	$100,000	24%	20%	55%
66%	$110,500	24%	23%	52%
61%	$150,000	24%	17%	58%

Made in United States
Cleveland, OH
05 November 2026

47664975R00029